DAILY HEALTH AND FITNESS

PERFECT HEALTH IN UNDER 45 MINUTES A DAY

SAM FURY

Illustrated by
OKIANG LUHUNG & NEIL GERMIO

Copyright SF Nonfiction Books © 2017

www.SFNonfictionBooks.com

All Rights Reserved
No part of this document may be reproduced without written consent from the author.

WARNINGS AND DISCLAIMERS

The information in this publication is made public for reference only.

Neither the author, publisher, nor anyone else involved in the production of this publication is responsible for how the reader uses the information or the result of his/her actions.

CONTENTS

Introduction   ix

Nutrition   1
Life Force   6

BODY CONDITIONING
SFP Super-burpee   11
Pull-ups   21

SFP YOGA STRETCH ROUTINE
Mountain Pose   25
Standing Backbend   27
Crescent Moon   28
Standing Forward Fold   29
Table Pose   30
Threading the Needle   31
Upward Dog   32
Downward Dog   33
Low Warrior   34
Half Prayer-Twist   35
Half-Pyramid   36
Extended Dog   37
Hero Pose   38
Lion Pose   39
Downward-Facing Frog   40
Staff Pose   41
Seated Forward Bend   42
Bound Angle   43
Seated Angle   45
Side Seated Angle   46
Joyful Baby   47
Wind-Relieving Pose   48
Supine Bound Angle   49
Corpse Pose   50

Yoga Stretch Routine Quick List	51
Yoga Nidra	52
References	56
Author Recommendations	57
About Sam Fury	59

THANKS FOR YOUR PURCHASE

Did you know you can get FREE chapters of any SF Nonfiction Book you want?

https://offers.SFNonfictionBooks.com/Free-Chapters

You will also be among the first to know of FREE review copies, discount offers, bonus content, and more.

Go to:

https://offers.SFNonfictionBooks.com/Free-Chapters

Thanks again for your support.

INTRODUCTION

Daily Health and Fitness is a complete body and mind health routine in four parts.

Do all four parts every day for optimal health.

1. **Nutrition.** What you put into your body matters—a lot
2. **Body Conditioning.** Two extremely efficient exercises to keep your whole body strong, including the awesome SFP Super-burpee.
3. **SFP Yoga Stretch Routine.** Stretch your whole body using this specially designed 15-minute yoga routine.
4. **Yoga Nidra.** A quick Yoga Nidra session as a form of daily meditation.

The nutrition guidelines provided here should be observed at all times. If you do the other three things back to back, they will take you less than 45 minutes. They can also be easily split up throughout the day to suit your schedule.

Be diligent in doing the above, and in under 45 minutes a day, you will be healthier in body and mind **than the majority of people on the planet!**

NUTRITION

These Survival Fitness Plan nutrition guidelines are easy to remember to stick with.

There are five major guidelines:

1. Fast for 16 hours a day.
2. Eat gut-healthy food.
3. Eat a plant-based, whole-foods diet.
4. Minimize refined sugar.
5. Minimize drug use.

16-Hour Fasting

This is intermittent fasting. There are several ways to do it, but I find this one way the best because it becomes part of your daily routine. It keeps things simple.

The stretch of time you choose depends on your lifestyle; all that matters is that it is 16 hours long. I like to fast between 8:00 p.m. and 12:00 p.m. the following day. All I'm doing is skipping breakfast.

During the fasting period, you can drink water, herbal tea, or black coffee. If you get hungry, try having a tablespoon of apple cider vinegar in a glass of water. A tablespoon of coconut oil is also good. You should consume these two things every day anyway. Both are good for your health.

Intermittent fasting has some great benefits. For example, it:

- Boosts the immune system
- Facilitates fat loss
- Improves longevity
- Lowers the risk of diabetes
- Helps you sleep better

- Slows aging
- Helps you think clearer

Eat Gut-Healthy Food

A healthy gut means a healthy mind and body. This is a scientific fact!

There are many food that are good for your guts. Kefir is one of the best, but if that's not your thing, then any fermented foods are good too. Apple cider vinegar, sauerkraut, kimchi, tempeh, miso, and pickles are all good examples.

You should also eat foods that are high in fiber, such as whole grains, beans, legumes, and whole fruits and veggies. Aim to get a good dose of high-fiber and fermented foods every day.

Plant-Based Whole Foods

What are whole foods? Here is a definition straight from Wikipedia:

"Whole foods are plant foods that are unprocessed and unrefined, or processed and refined as little as possible, before being consumed. Examples of whole foods include whole grains, tubers, legumes, fruits, vegetables."

https://en.wikipedia.org/wiki/Whole_food

As a bonus, eating a whole-foods diet will cut your food bill—by quite a lot, in some cases.

Anything made with white flour is not a whole food. This includes bread, cereals, crackers, granola bars, pasta, etc. You can still eat these things, but choose the non-white whole grain version instead. The same goes for white rice. Eat wild or brown rice instead. "Normal" potatoes are okay, but sweet potatoes are way better.

Here's a list of no white-flour foods:

https://www.livestrong.com/article/336585-list-of-no-white-flour-foods

Eat Less Refined Sugar

Refined sugar is poison, and is in many things. Here are some examples. The less of these things you eat, the healthier you'll be.

Processed food. Almost everything processed will have refined sugar in it. This covers most things that are not in the fresh-food section of the supermarket. The easiest way to know is by looking at the ingredients label.

Deep-fried foods. Most things that are deep-fried will also have refined sugar. Even if they don't, nothing deep-fried is good for you anyway.

Drinks. Drinks other than water and fresh herbal tea usually have quite a bit of sugar in them. Soft drinks are the worst. Clean water is the best drink you can have. Making it your main drink will flush your body of toxins. Aim to drink **at least** one liter every day. Herbal teas, either cold- or hot-brewed, are a good way to add a bit of flavor, as well as to get some extra benefits (such as aiding digestion and boosting your immunity).

Every morning when you wake, rinse your mouth out and then drink a couple of cups of water. It will assist rehydration from the night and stimulate your digestive system.

Minimize Drug Use

This includes alcohol, cigarettes, pharmaceuticals you don't need, and illicit drugs.

Of course, some drugs are worse than others. Smoking cigarettes, for example, is crazy. Drinking a little alcohol once in a while, not so bad.

Additional Healthy Eating Tips

Fruits. Fruits are great, but due to the large amount of fructose in them, consuming too many is bad for your teeth. Limit yourself to three servings a day.

Vegetables. You cannot eat too many vegetables. They should make up a big part of your diet. Local fruits and vegetables that are in season in your location are best.

Herbs. Not only do they make your food taste nicer, they are super healthy. Garlic, ginger, and chili are my favorites, and they are very cheap to buy and easy to grow. Garlic is crazy healthy.

Putting them in fresh salads or soups or steaming them are the best ways to prepare your vegetables. The next best is thing is to stir-fry or roast them. Stay away from deep-fried foods.

Bright or deep colors are best. Go for leafy greens, berries, red bell peppers, papaya, moringa, etc.

Wash all fruits and vegetables. Even organic fruits and vegetables can have poison sprayed on them. Ensure that you use water you would consider safe to drink.

Get a good variety. Different foods have different nutritional values. When it comes to fruit and vegetables, choose a variety of colors and types. This actually applies to all foods. Ensure you are consuming proteins, dairy, fruit, vegetables, complex carbohydrates, good fats, etc.

Proteins. Vegetarian proteins (tofu, eggs, beans, etc.) are best for health and other reasons. Failing that, go for fish (salmon is great) and lean meats (skinless chicken and lean beef are my favorites).

When you crave something sweet, go for dark chocolate. The higher the percentage of cocoa, the better. Raw honey is also great.

Benefits of Being Vegetarian

If you think you need meat for a balanced diet, you're incorrect. There are lots of replacement options, such as tofu, legumes, nuts, eggs, etc.

There are a few reasons I advocate vegetarianism:

- It's much healthier than most people realize.
- It removes the animal cruelty factor, especially with factory farming. It would be even better to go vegan.
- It saves money. In most cases, being vegetarian is cheaper than eating meat.

Here's a link to a documentary called *Mad Cowboy*. It's worth the watch:

www.youtube.com/watch?v=piZmH4gzyqs

LIFE FORCE

The life force is a non-physical essential energy that is present in all things in the universe, and the universe provides it in abundance for all.

Although the concept of the life force is rejected by modern science, the notion of it is present in most cultures, both Eastern and Western. Depending on where you are from, you may know it as chi, élan vital, gi, khi, ki, manitou, prana, ruah, qi, vitalism, etc.

In living creatures, this essential energy flows through the body. If it gets blocked, the blockage is manifested as illness and/or pain.

This means that any "sickness" you have, whether it be physical, mental, or emotional, is caused by blocked energy, and can be alleviated by releasing the blockage. It also means that sickness can be prevented by maintaining clear passages of this energy through the body. The simplest way to encourage and maintain the flow of this energy through the body is the breath.

Life Force and the Breath

Although every breath you take helps to circulate the life force throughout your body, taking full breaths is much more effective. Unfortunately, most people do not do so.

When you take the time to concentrate on proper breathing, it will promote better breathing even when you're not concentrating on it. It takes a cycle of nine breaths for the first breath to be exhaled from the body. I recommend doing four cycles of conscious breathing a day. These can be done all at once (36 breaths) or nine at a time at various times during the day.

Doing the Yoga Stretch Routine will cover 36 conscious breaths and then some. But you can do them whenever you want. The more, the better.

If you only want to do one thing a day to maintain your health, do conscious breathing.

Receiving the Breath

Get in a comfortable position. You can be lying, sitting, or standing. Completely exhale your whole breath. This is the effortful part.

Now just allow the inhale to come in naturally through your nose. There is no need to actively breathe in deeply. Just receive it. Over time, you'll notice that your breaths naturally get deeper.

As you breathe in and out it, may help to imagine the flow of energy carried by your breath. It comes up your back as you inhale, and down your front as you exhale.

Inhale all the goodness of a new positive energy, and exhale all the stale and negative.

Three-Part Breath

This is the breath you should do when actively practicing yoga, but when first learning it, you'll probably just want to do it from a sitting or lying position.

Breathe in long and deep through your nose. First, feel it enter your lower belly, then your lower chest/rib cage, and finally your lower throat/ the top of your sternum. Feel the clear, positive energies of happiness and love come up from your toes to your head.

When you are ready, exhale fully through your nose, feeling the breath leave in the opposite order from the one it came in— that is, first from your sternum, then from your chest, and finally from your belly. Release all negative energy and tension out of your body, from your head to your toes. Continue to breathe in and out like this, smoothly and continuously.

When you first start to practice this type of breathing, it may help to put your hands on each of the three areas (belly, chest, and sternum) as you do it. You can also try just breathing into each area on its own.

BODY CONDITIONING

This section describes two exercises designed to keep your physical body strong in the most efficient way.

5 SFP super-burpees is the bare minimum of daily exercise.

The ideal daily conditioning routine is:

- 10 SFP super-burpees
- 10 pull-ups

SFP SUPER-BURPEE

The Survival Fitness Plan (SFP) super-burpee is an extremely efficient exercise that acts as a warm-up, light stretch, and full-body muscle conditioning workout all in one.

When several super-burpees are done properly and in succession, they also serve to fill the body with life force, as well as to give a cardiovascular workout. Furthermore, the exercise has been tweaked over time to give additional benefits in relation to SFP fight and flight activities such as parkour and self-defense.

Here is a list of the main benefits gained from the SFP super-burpee:

- Balance
- Cardiovascular workout
- Circulation of life force
- Coordination
- Explosiveness
- Improved bodily function (digestion, respiration, etc.)
- Flexibility
- Muscle conditioning
- Hang time (the ability to stay airborne)
- Striking strength and speed
- Warm-up

I highly recommended doing **at least** five SFP super-burpees every morning to ready your body for the day. One SFP super-burpee takes less than 10 seconds.

Even if you only have one minute to spare for exercise, you have time to do SFP super-burpees!

I also recommend doing SFP super-burpees as a general warm-up before any vigorous exercise, such as SFP Fight and Flight training.

The SFP super-burpee is made up of five separate exercises, each of which has been specifically chosen and tweaked to provide the most benefit in relation to the Survival Fitness Plan.

Jumping squats: Jumping squats develop leg strength, core strength, explosiveness, soft landing skills, jumping ability, and hang-time.

Finger-tip push-ups: Finger-tip push-ups increase finger strength and grip, increase striking power, and improve all-over body conditioning.

Clapping push-ups: These are great for increasing striking power and all-over body conditioning. The clapping part really improves explosiveness, which is awesome for speed and power. The push-up also condition your hands for the palm-heel strike which is preferred over a fist in SFP Self-Defense training.

Hindu Push-ups: Hindu push-ups use the downward dog and the upward dog (yoga poses) which are beneficial for your:

- Brain (stimulates)
- Breathing (chest)
- Concentration
- Eyesight
- Hearing
- Kidneys
- Memory
- Nervous system
- Spine
- Whole-body strengthening

Brazilians: Brazilians mainly contribute to cardiovascular workout and hip flexibility, but they also increase core strength and work the lower abdominals.

If you are unable to do a full SFP super-burpee, you can build yourself up to them by doing each individual exercise separately.

Once you can do each 10 repetitions of each individual exercise, you should be strong enough to put them together into an SFP super-burpee.

The first SFP super-burpee you do for the day (or when warming up for exercise) must be done slowly and with much purpose.

If you try to do fast super-burpees straight away, your chances of injury will greatly increase. Doing the first one very well will warm up and stretch your body. After that, you can gradually increase speed with the second and third repetitions until you are going full-speed for as many reps as you can handle.

Note: If you have any injuries, please leave out any part of the SFP super-burpee that may aggravate them.

The following is a detailed explanation of how to do a full SFP super-burpee as if it's the first one.

Jumping Squat

Stand straight, with your feet shoulder-width apart.

As you breathe in, squat down as low as you can. Keep your back straight and come up on your toes as you squat down. Put your arms out to your front. This will help you keep your back straight.

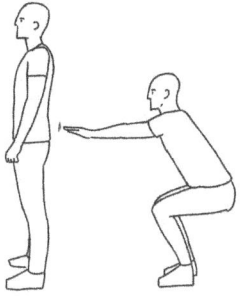

Spring up as you exhale, and jump as high as you can. Tuck your legs up as high as possible on the outside of your elbows. Try to keep your back straight. This is actually a box jump.

Land as softly as you can, and adopt a crouching squat position.

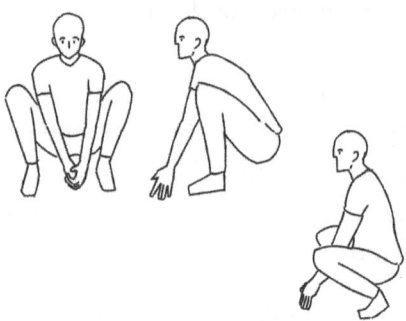

Note: If you can't do a jumping squat, you can build up to one by doing regular squats first. Just do as explained above, but without the jump.

Finger-tip push-up

From the squat position, as you inhale, place your fingertips firmly on the ground next to your feet and shoot both your legs behind you, so you're in the standard up position for a push-up, with the exception of being on your fingertips.

Ensure that your elbows are as close to your torso as possible, and that they are facing back towards your feet. This is so you target the muscles used for striking.

Grip the floor with your fingers, as if you're trying to rip a chunk out of the ground. Keep this grip throughout the push-up.

As you inhale, lower your chest until your arms are at a 90° angle at the elbow.

Push back up as fast as possible to the up position.

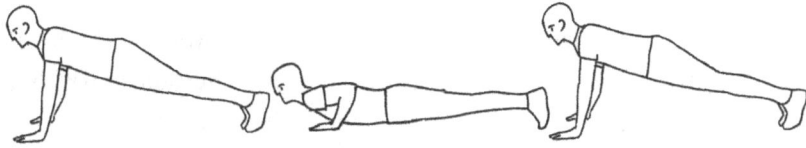

Clapping Push-up

Lower your chest again as you inhale.

This time, as you exhale, push up hard enough for you to be able to get your hands off the ground and clap.

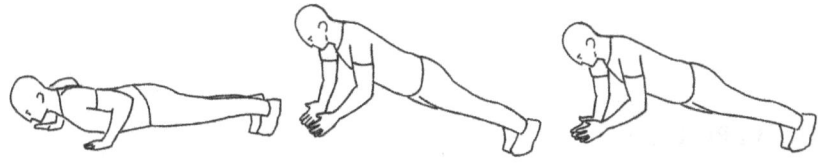

Aim to land on the palms of your hands as softly as possible and then return to the up position of the push-up.

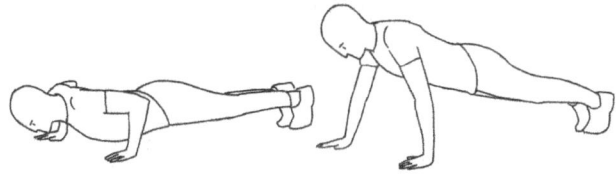

Note: If you can't do either of these push-ups, work your way up to them with normal push-ups. Next, do finger-tip pushups, and then clapping pushups.

If you can't yet do a normal push-up, work your way up to it first by just lying on your stomach and pushing up. Push on the ground for 10 seconds, and then rest. This is one rep. Do three sets of three reps every day. Eventually you'll be able to do a push-up. Once you can do 10 normal push-ups, try for fingertip push-ups.

It will help to do finger-strengthening exercises as well. A simple and very effective one is to place your fingertips together and push them against each other for as long as you can. Do it every day until you are able to do fingertip push-ups.

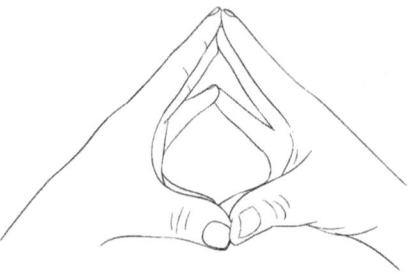

Hindu Push-up

From the up position of the push-up, breathe in and go into downward dog. If this is your first SFP super-burpee, spend a couple of breaths here to stretch your body. Go up on each foot to stretch your legs and really extend your upper body.

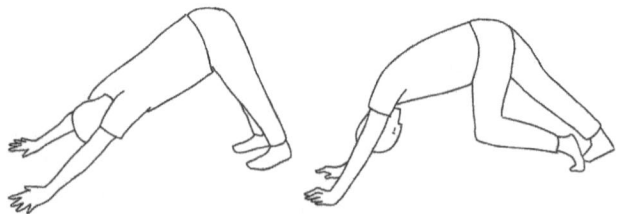

As you breathe out, sweep down in a circular arc motion into upward dog.

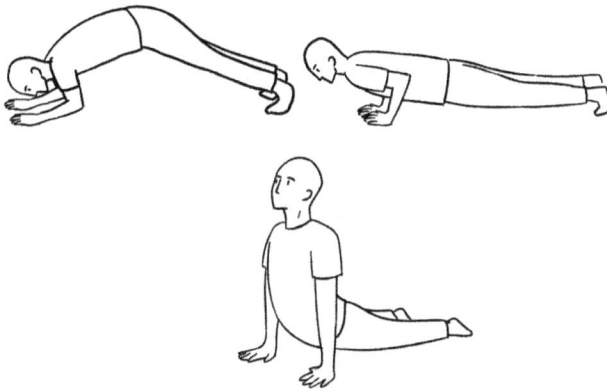

Again, if this is your first SFP super-burpee, spend a couple of breaths here to stretch your body.

Really arch your back and look high above. Move your neck from side to side and stretch out your arms, back, and upper thighs. When you're ready, inhale and return to the up position of the push-up.

Brazilians

As you exhale, bring your right knee to your left elbow and then back. Then bring your left knee to your right elbow. This is one rep of a Brazilian.

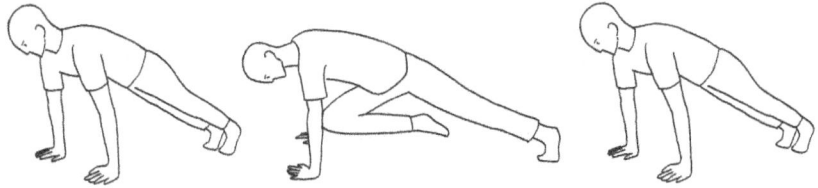

Jump back into a squat and then stand up straight.

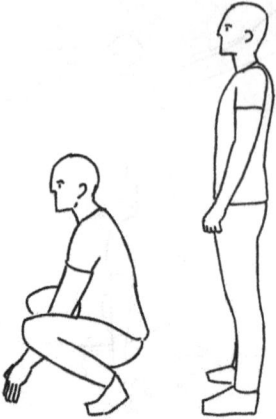

This completes one repetition of an SFP super-burpee.

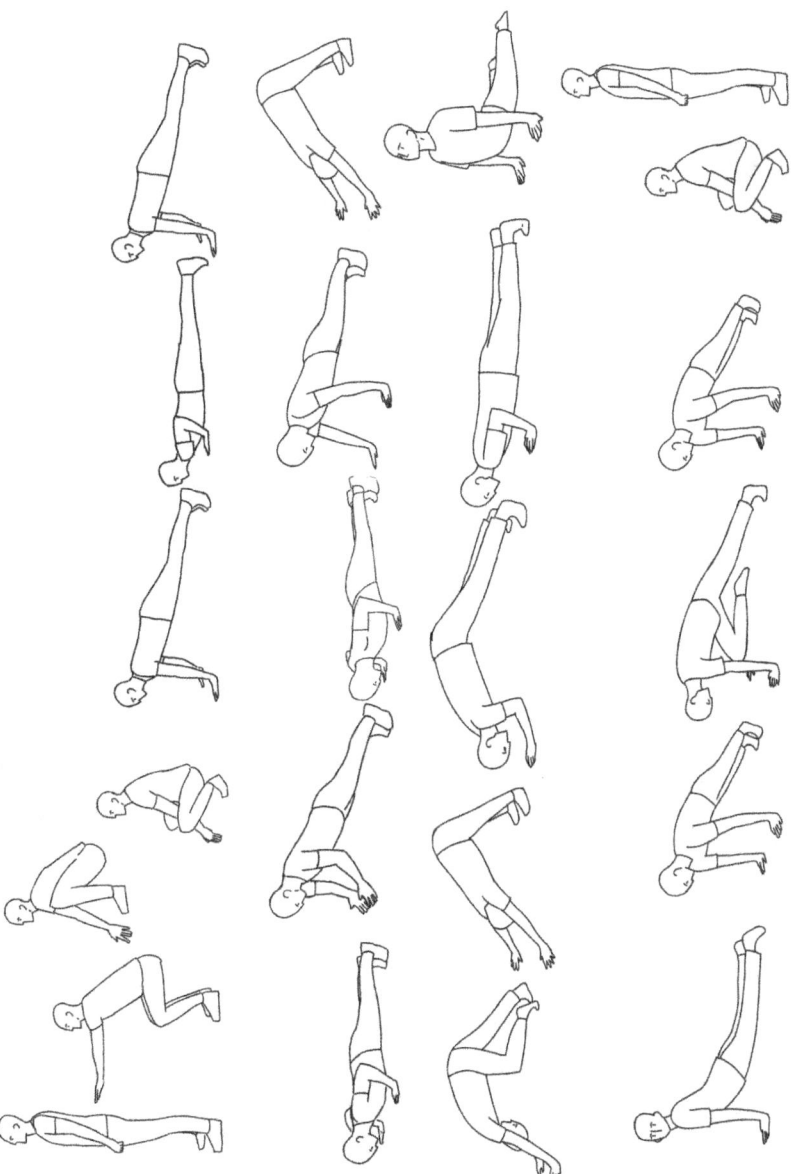

A complete SFP super-burpee

Related Chapters:

- Life Force
- Upward Dog
- Downward Dog

PULL-UPS

Being able to pull yourself up is an extremely useful skill, and the best way to condition yourself to do so is with the classic pull-up.

The pull-up is an especially useful exercise for the Survival Fitness Plan. It helps you build strength for parkour wall-climbs and, eventually, muscle-ups.

The following description is an excerpt from the book *Essential Parkour* by Sam Fury.

www.SFNonfictionBooks.com/Essential-Parkour

*** Start of Excerpt ***

Pull-ups are an excellent all-body exercise.

Grab the bar with a grip slightly wider than shoulder-width apart and with your palms facing away from you.

Let yourself hang all the way down.

Pull yourself up by pulling your shoulder blades down and together. Keep your chest up and pull up until your chin is above the bar. Touch your chest to it.

As you are pulling up, keep your body in a vertical line. Do not swing. Concentrate on isolating your back and biceps.

Pause at the top, and then lower yourself back down into the hanging position.

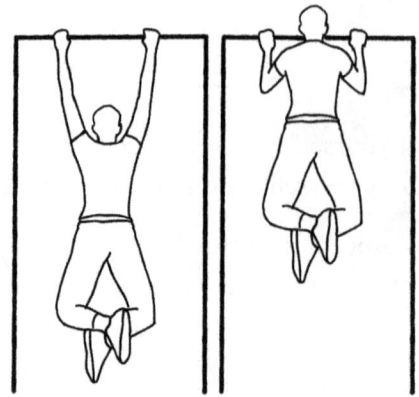

SFP YOGA STRETCH ROUTINE

The SFP yoga cool-down is a whole body stretch which also gives the many other benefits of yoga. Balance, a calm mind, coordination, core strength, development of chi, flexibility, etc.

This yoga cool-down is approximately 15 minutes long if you stay in each pose for two to three breaths. The longer you stay in each pose for, the more beneficial it is, so go longer than 15 minutes if you want.

Whilst doing this routine it is important to move slowly and use conscious breathing.

Although all the poses used in this book are considered basic ones, you may find some of them challenging when you're first starting.

Adjust them to your comfort level and work your way up. Hold each pose to the point where you can feel a good stretch, but not pain.

You will probably notice your breath shorten if you try to force your body too much. When this happens, just back off a little and refocus on your breathing. If you do find yourself in a painful position, back out of it slowly to avoid injury.

Note: If you are planning to do more physical exercise as part of this routine, do it after conditioning and before this yoga stretch routine.

The information in this section is from the book *Curing Yoga* by Aventuras De Viaje.

www.SFNonfictionBooks.com/Curing-Yoga

MOUNTAIN POSE

Avoid this if you have a shoulder injury.

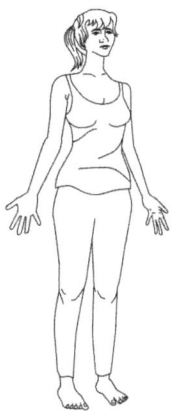

Stand with your feet parallel and either together or hip-width apart.

Spread your toes wide and balance your weight evenly and centrally over each foot.

Pull up your kneecaps and tense your thighs. Keep your legs straight, but do not lock your knees. Ensure your hips are directly over your ankles.

As you inhale, lengthen your spine so that the crown of your head goes straight up towards the sky.

When you exhale, drop your shoulders and stretch your fingertips towards the ground, whilst still extending your head upwards. At the same time, gently push your chest straight ahead.

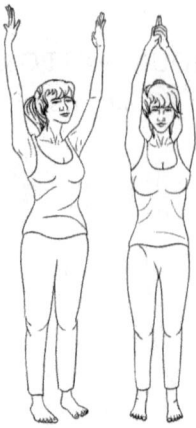

While continuing to stretch your fingertips, inhale and bring your arms up above your head to reach for the sky, palms facing each other.

As you exhale, relax your shoulders, but continue to stretch your crown and fingers towards the sky. An alternative position is to interlace your fingers with your index fingers pointing up.

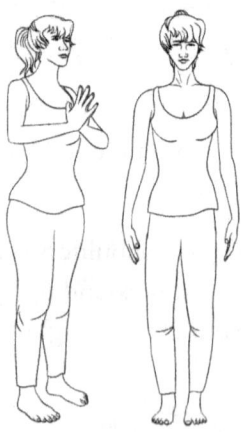

When you're ready, exhale and bring your palms together in front of your chest in a prayer position. Take a breath, and allow your hands to drop to your sides on the exhale.

STANDING BACKBEND

Avoid this if you have a back, hip, and/or neck injury.

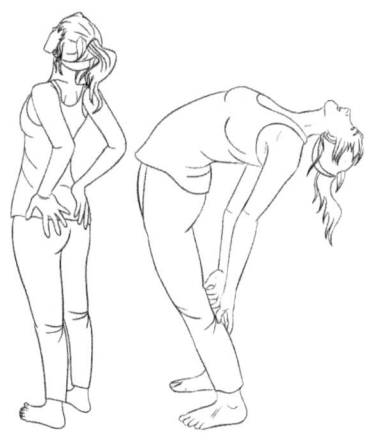

Stand with your feet parallel and hip-width apart.

As you breathe in, place the palms of your hands on your lower back (sacrum) with your fingers pointing to the ground.

Squeeze your buttocks and thighs tightly together, pull up your kneecaps, and press into your feet.

Exhale and press your hips forward as you arch your back.

You can either look straight ahead or allow your head to drop all the way back.

Increase the stretch by walking your hands down the back of your legs.

When you're ready, slowly come back to a standing position with your hands by your sides.

CRESCENT MOON

Avoid this if you have a back, hip, and/or shoulder injury.

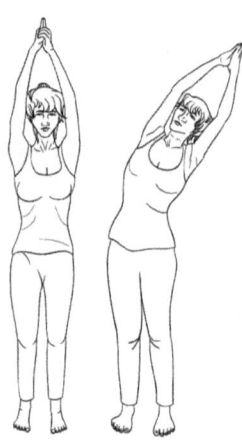

Stand with your feet parallel and either together or hip-width apart.

While inhaling, join your hands together above your head with your fingers interlaced and your index fingers pointing to the sky.

As you exhale, push your left hip out to the side and arch to your left. Keep your body strong and lengthened.

Inhale as you return to the position, with your fingers interlaced and your index fingers pointing to the sky. Repeat it on your other side.

STANDING FORWARD FOLD

Avoid this if you have a back, hip, leg, and/or shoulder injury.

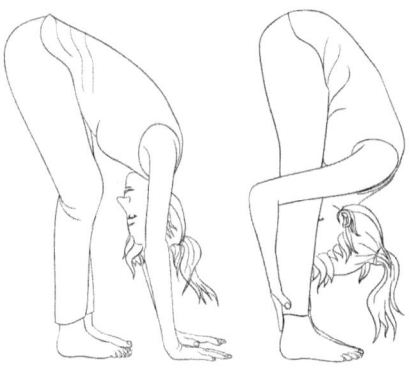

Stand with your feet parallel and either together or hip-width apart.

Exhale and bring your head to your knees, with your palms flat on the floor.

Stretch your spine by pulling your head down while pushing your hips up. Bend your knees if you need to, but aim to be able to do it with straight legs. Press your belly into your thighs when inhaling.

For a deeper stretch, hold the back of your calves and pull your head closer to your legs.

TABLE POSE
Avoid this if you have a knee and/or wrist injury.

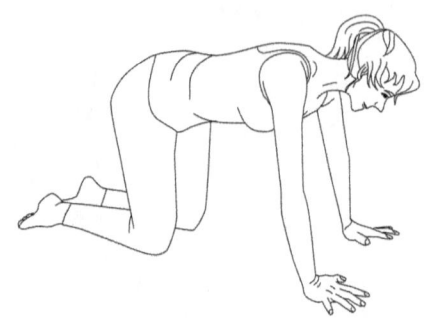

As you inhale, place your hands and knees on the floor, with your palms directly underneath your shoulders and fingers facing forward.

Ensure your knees are shoulder-width apart and your feet are directly behind them, with the tops of your feet and toes on the floor.

Look at the ground between your hands and press down into your palms.

Have your back flat and exhale while lengthening your spine by pressing the crown of your head forward and your tailbone back.

THREADING THE NEEDLE

Avoid this if you have a knee, neck, and/or shoulder injury.

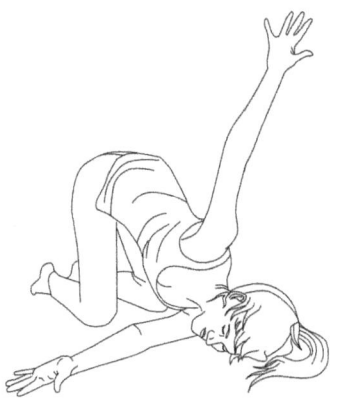

Place your hands and knees on the floor, with your palms directly underneath your shoulders and fingers facing forward. Your knees are shoulder-width apart and your feet are directly behind them. Have your back flat.

As you exhale, slide your right hand between your left knee and left hand until your right shoulder and the side of your head are resting on the floor.

Inhale and reach towards the sky with your left hand. Find where you get the deepest stretch and stay there, reaching out with your fingers.

When you're ready, exhale as you bring your hand back to the floor and then inhale to readopt your starting position.

Repeat on your left side.

UPWARD DOG

Avoid if you have an arm, back, hip, and/or shoulder injury, have had recent abdominal surgery, and/or are pregnant.

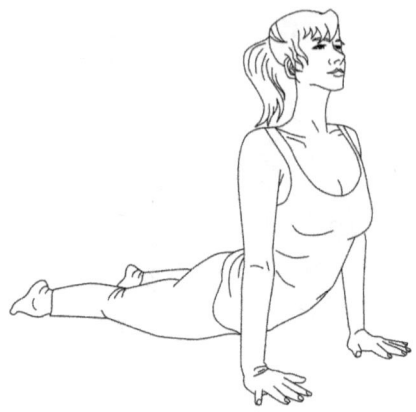

Place your hands and knees on the floor, with your palms directly underneath your shoulders and fingers facing forward. Your knees are shoulder-width apart and your feet are directly behind them. Have your back flat.

Drop your hips forward towards the ground as you press your palms down into the floor.

Press your chest forward as you drop your shoulders down and back.

Push the crown of your head towards the ceiling.

As you inhale, press the tops of your feet into the ground to lift your legs off the floor. Only the tops of your feet and your hands should touch the ground. Press all of your toenails firmly into the floor.

DOWNWARD DOG

Avoid this if you have an arm, back, hip, and/or shoulder injury, and/or unmediated high blood pressure.

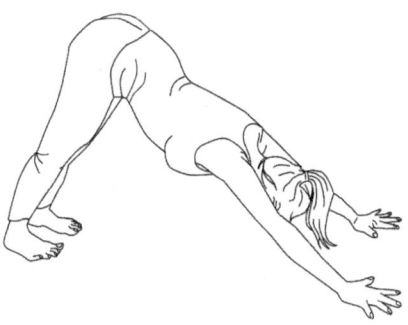

Place your hands and knees on the floor, with your palms directly underneath your shoulders and fingers facing forward. Your knees are shoulder-width apart and your feet are directly behind them. Have your back flat.

As you inhale, tuck in your toes so you are on the balls of your feet. Keep your palms shoulder width apart and spread your fingers apart, with your middle fingers facing forward.

Press into your hands and lift your hips towards the sky.

Push your hips up and back. Your chest should move towards your thighs. Keep your arms straight, but don't lock your elbows.

Keep your spine straight as you lift up through your tailbone.

Stretch the backs of your legs by pressing your heels to the floor. Keep your back flat. Your legs should be straight (knees not locked) or with a small bend at the knees.

Let your head dangle freely.

LOW WARRIOR
Avoid this if you have an ankle, arm, hip, and/or shoulder injury.

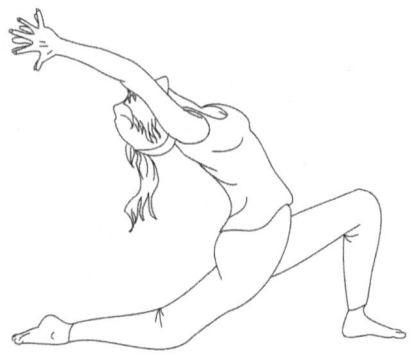

Place your hands and knees on the floor, with your palms directly underneath your shoulders and fingers facing forward. Your knees are shoulder-width apart and your feet are directly behind them. Have your back flat.

Step your right foot forward, placing it in between your hands. Your knee should be directly over your ankle.

Ensure your left knee and left and right feet are firmly on the ground, and then place your hands on your right knee.

Straighten your arms and bring your torso back. Do not lock your elbows.

Relax your shoulders and stick your chest out by bringing your shoulder blades towards each other.

As you inhale, raise your arms over your head with your palms facing each other and arch your back as you look up to the sky. If this is difficult, then you can keep your hands on your bent knee.

When you're ready, exhale as you bring your palms back to the floor on either side of your right foot.

HALF PRAYER-TWIST

Avoid this if you have a back, hip, knee, and/or shoulder injury.

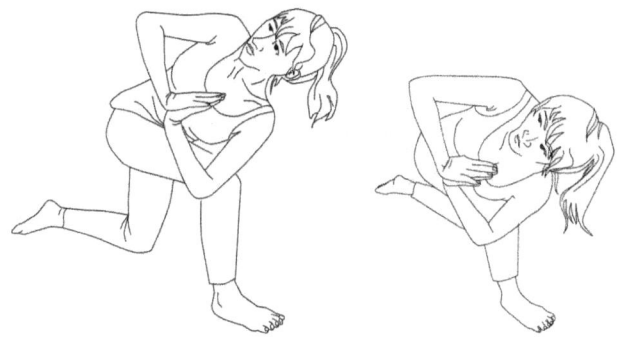

Adopt a low lunge position with your right foot forward and your left lower leg flat on the ground. Place your palms on the floor, one on each side of your front foot.

As you inhale, bring your torso up and place your hands together in a prayer position.

Place your left elbow to the outside of your right knee and use your arms to press your left shoulder up and back. Feel it twist your upper back.

Ensure your palms remain in the center of your chest with your fingers pointing towards your throat.

You can either look straight ahead or up towards the sky.

When you're ready, exhale as you bring your palms back to the floor, one on each side of your left foot.

HALF-PYRAMID

Avoid this if you have a knee and/or leg injury.

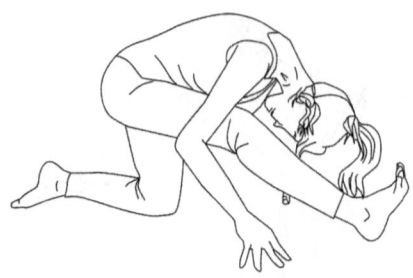

Adopt a low lunge position with your right foot forward and your left lower leg flat on the ground.

While exhaling, straighten your right leg as you press your hips back towards your left heel.

Round your spine and lift your toes to the sky as you push your forehead into your right knee. Walk your hands back towards you to support your torso. Relax your elbows, face, neck, and shoulders.

When you're ready, inhale and bend your right knee back over your ankle, and then exhale and bring your right knee back next to your left one.

EXTENDED DOG

Avoid this if you have an arm, back, knee, and/or shoulder injury.

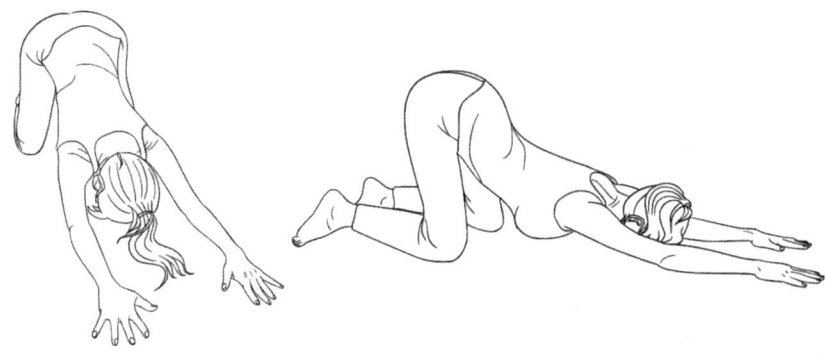

Place your hands and knees on the floor, with your palms directly underneath your shoulders and fingers facing forward. Your knees are shoulder-width apart and your feet are directly behind them. Have your back flat.

As you inhale, push your tailbone towards the sky then exhale and lower your forehead to the floor by sliding your hands forward. Ensure you keep your hips lifted over your knees.

Arch the middle of your back by allowing your chest to sink towards the floor.

Deepen the stretch by straightening your arms, lifting your elbows off the floor, and bringing your hips back. Try not to let your hands slide while you do this.

Place your chin on the ground to stretch your neck.

When you're ready, inhale and return to your starting position.

HERO POSE
Avoid this if you have a knee injury.

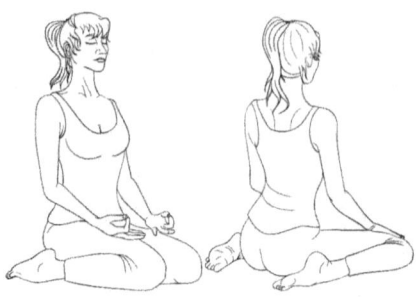

Kneel on the ground with your knees together and your feet hip-width apart. Sit with your bum on the ground and your heels on the outside of your hips. If this is too difficult, you can sit on your heels.

Place your hands on your knees. Your palms can face up or down.

Lengthen your torso by reaching the crown of your head to the sky.

Push your lower legs into the ground, drop your shoulders, and press your chest forward.

Relax your belly, face, jaw, and tongue.

Hero pose is an excellent pose for rest and/or meditation.

LION POSE

Avoid this if you have a face, knee, neck, and/or tongue injury.

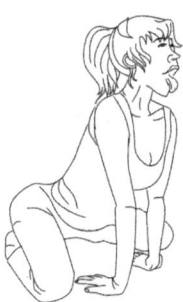

Kneel on the ground with your knees together and your feet hip-width apart. Sit with your bum on the ground and your heels on the outside of your hips.

Bring your feet together and spread your knees as wide as you comfortably can.

Sit on your heels.

Inhale and lengthen your spine by stretching the crown of your head towards the sky.

Bring your palms to the floor in between your knees, with your fingers facing your body.

Arch your spine, stick your tongue out, and exhale ferociously via your mouth.

Repeat this a few times.

DOWNWARD-FACING FROG

Avoid this if you have a knee, hip, and/or leg injury.

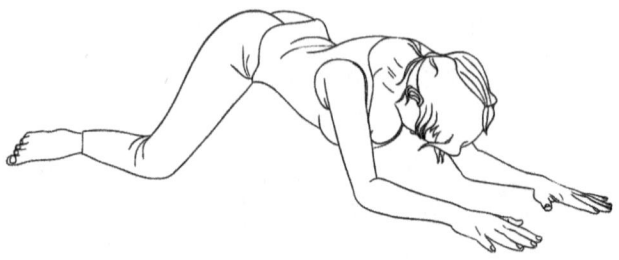

Kneel on the ground with your knees together and your feet hip-width apart. Sit with your bum on the ground and your heels on the outside of your hips.

Spread your knees as wide as you comfortably can and align your feet so that they are directly behind them—that is, with your right foot behind your right knee and your left foot behind your left knee.

Turn your feet outwards so your toes are facing away from your body.

Place your elbows, forearms, and palms flat on the floor.

Exhale as you push your hips back.

STAFF POSE

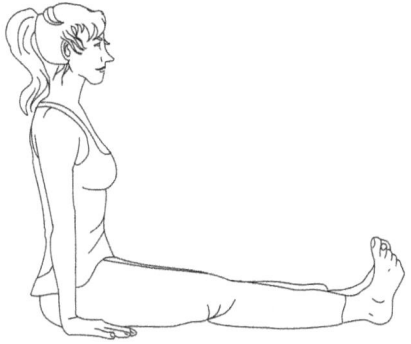

Start in a seated position with your legs extended straight out in front of you. Place your hands beside your hips with your fingers pointed forward.

Lengthen your spine by pressing your hip bones down while pushing the crown of your head towards the sky. Use your arms for support as you push your chest forward and lower your shoulders.

Pull your toes towards your head as you push your heels away from you.

SEATED FORWARD BEND
Avoid this if you have an ankle, arm, hip, and/or shoulder injury.

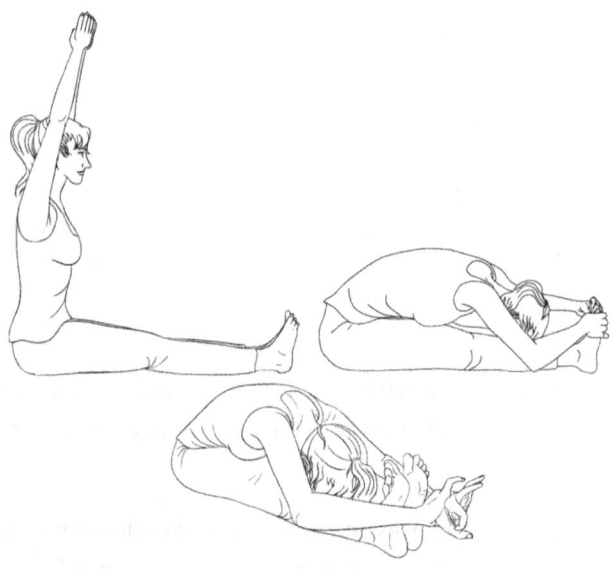

Start in a seated position with your legs extended straight out in front of you. Inhale and raise your arms up to the sky, with your palms facing each other. Lengthen your torso through your fingers and the crown of your head.

As you exhale, bend at the hips, lowering your upper body to your legs. Grab your ankles, feet, or toes.

Push out through your heels as you pull your toes back towards you.

You can use your arms to pull yourself closer to your legs. If you have more flexibility, reach your hands in front of your feet. If you're having difficulties, bend your knees enough so that you can reach your feet and place your head on your knees.

When you're ready, slowly roll up your spine back into the seated position.

BOUND ANGLE

Avoid this if you have a hip and/or knee injury.

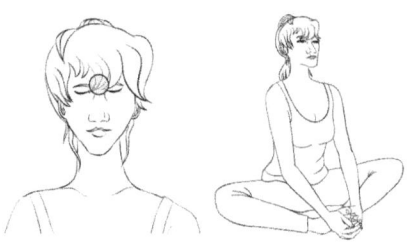

Start in a seated position with your legs extended straight out in front of you.

Bend your legs to bring the bottoms of your feet together. Your knees should bend outwards.

Hold onto your toes by lacing your fingers around them.

As you inhale, stretch the crown of your head up towards the sky while pushing your hips down. Push your chest forward and relax your shoulders down.

Close your eyes and look to your third eye (behind the middle of your forehead).

As you exhale, push your knees to the ground and gently pull your torso forward. Ensure you're keeping your chest open and your back flat.

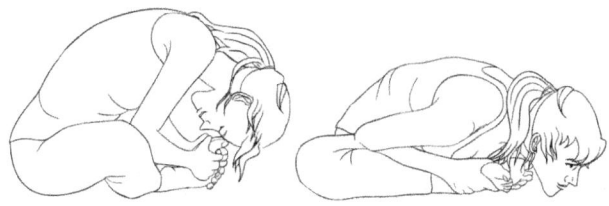

For a deeper stretch, pull your forehead or chest towards your feet. When you're ready, return to staff pose.

Related Chapters:

- Staff Pose

SEATED ANGLE

Avoid this if you have an arm, hip, knee, and/or shoulder injury.

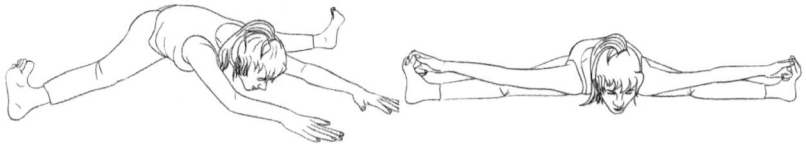

Start in a seated position with your legs extended straight out in front of you.

As you inhale, spread your legs out as wide as comfortable.

Ensure your knees and toes are pointing up and reach through your fingers up to the sky.

Exhale as you lower your palms to the floor.

Deepen the stretch by walking your hands forward. Stay focused on keeping your spine long. You could also hold your big toes and use them to help pull your torso down.

When you're ready, inhale and slowly walk your hands in as you roll back your spine until you finish with a straight back.

SIDE SEATED ANGLE
Avoid if you have a hip, leg, and/or lower back injury.

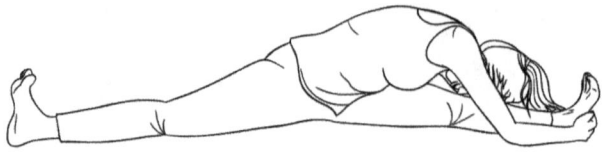

Start in a seated position with your legs spread your legs out as wide as comfortable.

Turn to face your right foot by twisting at your waist.

Walk your hands towards your right foot as you exhale. Try to reach your forehead to your knee and hold your right ankle or foot if you are able.

Relax your shoulders and neck and then increase the stretch by pressing your heel out while pulling your toes back towards yourself.

When you're ready, return to center with your back straight and then do the same thing on your left side.

JOYFUL BABY

Avoid this if you have a leg, neck, and/or shoulder injury.

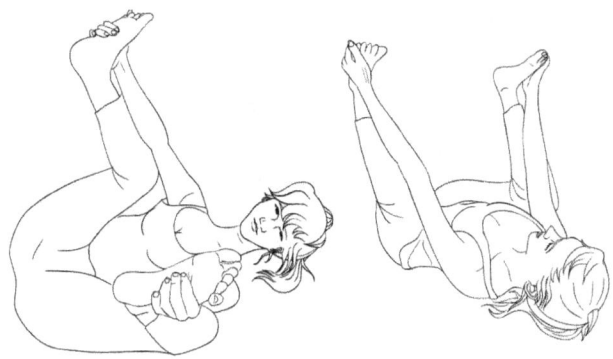

Lie flat on your back on the floor.

As you inhale, bring your knees to your chest.

Weave your arms through the inside of your knees and hold onto the pinkie-toe sides of your feet with your hands.

Keep your head on the ground and tuck your chin to your chest.

Push your heels up to the sky as you pull back with your arms. At the same time, press the back of your neck, shoulders, sacrum, and tailbone to the floor.

Open your legs wider for a deeper hip stretch.

When you're ready, exhale and slowly roll your spine back to the ground until you're lying flat again.

WIND-RELIEVING POSE

Avoid this if you have a hernia and/or have had recent abdominal surgery.

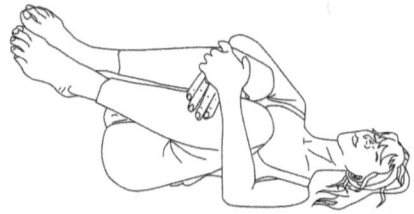

Lie flat on your back on the floor.

As you inhale, bring both knees up to your chest.

Hug your knees and hold onto the elbows, forearms, fingers, or wrists of your opposite arm (that is, hold your right arm with your left hand, and vice versa).

Keep your head on the floor while tucking your chin to your chest.

Pull your knees to your chest as you press the back of your neck, shoulders, sacrum, and tailbone to the floor. Relax your feet, hips, and legs.

Inhale deeply into your belly and press it against your thighs as you do so.

When you're ready, exhale and relax all your limbs to the ground so you are lying flat again.

SUPINE BOUND ANGLE

Avoid this if you have a hip and/or shoulder injury.

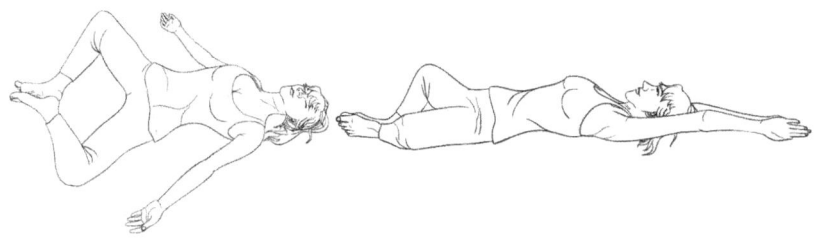

Lie flat on your back on the floor. Bend your legs to bring the bottoms of your feet together.

Your knees should face out just like in bound angle, but lying down. Allow your knees to drop to the ground.

You can rest your hands on your thighs to "encourage" them, but don't push down.

As you inhale, slide your arms on the ground over your head until your palms are together. Cross your thumbs.

When you're ready, exhale as you return to a lying position.

Related Chapters:

- Bound Angle

CORPSE POSE

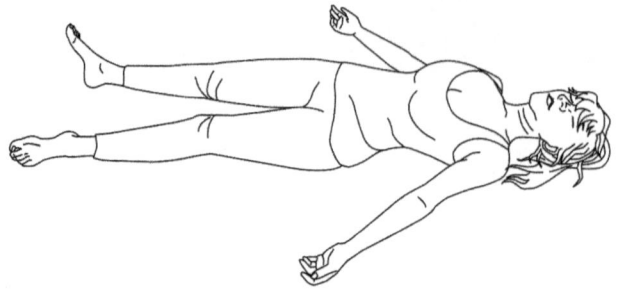

Lie flat on your back on the floor. You can place a pillow under your head if you want.

Keep your head straight; don't let it fall to the side.

Draw your shoulder blades down and open your chest towards your chin.

Have your arms at a comfortable distance from your body, with your palms facing up. Completely relax your arms and fingers.

Lift and extend your buttocks to your heels so that your whole sacrum rests on the floor.

Keep your abdomen soft and relaxed.

Slowly stretch your legs out straight, one at the time. Allow them to roll out to the side from the hips to the feet. Check that your body is in a straight line and you are resting evenly on the left and right sides.

Once you're comfortable, stay perfectly still and quiet and be aware of your body relaxing deeper into the floor. Allow your eyes to rest completely so they sink deeper towards the back of the skull. Relax your whole face and body. Be aware of your breath, quiet and soft.

Yoga Cool-Down and Stretch Routine Quick-List

Transitional poses are those with *asterisks.

1. Mountain
2. Standing backbend
3. Crescent moon
4. Standing forward fold
5. Table
6. Threading the needle left
7. *Table
8. Threading the needle right
9. *Table
10. Upward dog
11. Downward dog
12. *Table
13. Low warrior left
14. Half prayer twist left
15. Half pyramid left
16. *Table
17. Low warrior right
18. Half prayer twist right
19. Half pyramid right
20. *Table
21. Extended dog
22. *Table
23. Hero
24. Lion
25. Downward frog
26. Staff
27. Seated forward bend
28. *Staff
29. Bound angle
30. *Staff
31. Seated angle
32. Side seated angle left
33. *Seated angle
34. Side seated angle right
35. *Seated angle
36. *Staff
37. Joyful baby
38. Wind relieving
39. Supine bound angle
40. Corpse

The longer you stay in each pose, the more beneficial it is, so go longer than 15 minutes if you want.

Other than the first time they appear, table pose, staff pose, and seated angle are transitional poses (marked with *asterisks). When doing a 15-minute routine, only stay in them for a few seconds.

YOGA NIDRA

Yoga Nidra is a form of guided meditation that has many health benefits. You can guide yourself, but the easiest way to do it is to listen to a Yoga Nidra practice and do what the instructor says.

The Survival Fitness Plan in to do **at least** ten minutes of Yoga Nidra immediately following the yoga cool-down.

Yoga Nidra is used in the Survival Fitness Plan because it is guided meditation, which makes it relatively easy to do, especially for beginners. If you use other forms of mediation that you enjoy, then feel free to stick to them. The main thing is that you do some sort meditation.

For best results, find a place where your body can be comfortable and you can practice undisturbed. It shouldn't be too hot or cold. Put on some soothing background music if you want.

It is best not to do Yoga Nidra in bed, because you'll be more likely to fall asleep. A yoga mat on the floor is ideal.

Yoga Nidra is a conscious practice.

Note: Ten minutes is a very short time to do Yoga Nidra. If you can spare the extra time, you can download some really good Yoga Nidra practices for free at:

YogaNidraNetwork.org/downloads.

Lie in Corpse Pose

Lie in corpse pose, as previously explained.

Corpse pose, a.k.a. shavasana, is a yoga pose used at the end of almost every yoga practice. Going straight from your yoga practice to Yoga Nidra is ideal and is (in my opinion) most likely the intention of the ones who created it.

Yoga Nidra can also be done from a sitting position if lying down is inappropriate.

Close your eyes.

Notice Your Breath

Notice your breathing. Feel your lungs filling with air, your stomach expanding, and then deflating.

Imagine a light around your body expanding and contracting as you breathe in and out. Feel the energy coursing through your body.

Use Your Senses

Notice each of your senses individually.

What sounds do you hear? Near, far, inside, outside.

What smells can you smell? Take small sniffs, like a dog does.

Taste the air.

Feel your body supported on the floor. Which parts of your body are touching?

What can you see with your eyes closed? Does the light make shapes on your eyelids?

Repeat Your Mantra

Your mantra is a short sentence stating your intentions. It's kind of like an affirmation. It may be an overall statement of health, relaxation, etc., or it may be a visualization of something you want to achieve.

Whatever it is, repeat it mentally three times. Try to feel how you would feel if the visualization was realized.

One I use often is "My entire being is completely relaxed and at one with the universe."

Scan Your Body

This is where you consciously relax each part of your body.

Mentally go through your body. Bring your attention to and relax each part. You can be very detailed about this, or just do large areas. I start from the top of my head and work my way down. Sometimes I even do internal organs.

After you have relaxed smaller body parts, relax whole sections. For example, relax your shoulder, upper arm, bicep, elbow, forearm, hand, fingers, and then your whole arm. At the end, relax your whole body as one.

Awaken the Body

The last step is to slowly deepen your breath and start to move your fingers and toes, then your hands and feet.

In your own time, stretch your body out in whatever way feels right. Open your eyes when you're ready.

When you're done stretching, gently hug your knees (wind-relieving pose). Fall to your right side and then gently sit up. Take a moment to reflect on the practice, and then go about your day.

Related Chapters:

- Wind-Relieving Pose
- Corpse Pose

THANKS FOR READING

Dear reader,

Thank you for reading *Daily Health and Fitness*.

If you enjoyed this book, please leave a review where you bought it. It helps more than most people think.

Don't forget your FREE book chapters!

You will also be among the first to know of FREE review copies, discount offers, bonus content, and more.

Go to:

https://offers.SFNonfictionBooks.com/Free-Chapters

Thanks again for your support.

REFERENCES

Burmeister, A. Monte, T. (1997). *The Touch of Healing: Energizing the Body, Mind, and Spirit With Jin Shin Jyutsu*. Bantam.

Cherng, W. (2014). *Daoist Meditation: The Purification of the Heart Method of Meditation and Discourse on Sitting and Forgetting.* Singing Dragon.

Dalai Lama. (2009). *The Art of Happiness: A Handbook for Living.* Hachette.

DK Publishing. (2011). *Yoga for a New You.* DK.

Ferriss, T. (2010). *The 4-Hour Body.* Harmony.

Fury, M. (2011). *The Definitive Guide To Burning Fat and Building Muscle.* CelebrityPress.

Gibbs, B. Hall, D. Smith, J.(2013). *The Complete Guide To Yoga: The essential guide to yoga for all the family with 800 step-by-step practical photographs* . Southwater.

Ming, S. (2006). *The Shaolin Workout: 28 Days to Transforming Your Body and Soul the Warrior's Way.* Rodale Books.

Page, D. (2015). Yoga for Regular Guys: The Best Damn Workout On The Planet!. Authorscape.

AUTHOR RECOMMENDATIONS

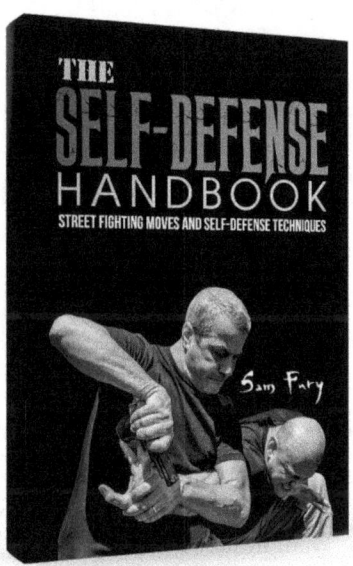

Teach Yourself Self-Defense!

This is the only self-defense training manual you need, because these are the best street fighting moves around.

Get it now.

www.SFNonfictionBooks.com/Self-Defense-Handbook

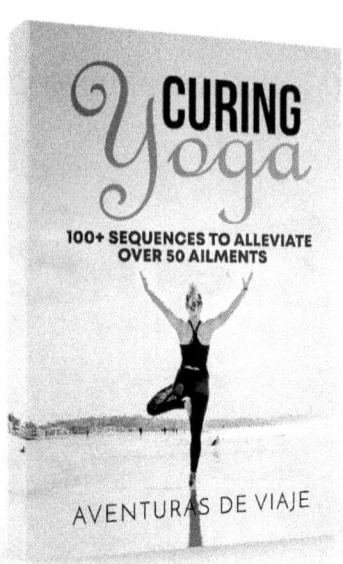

Discover How to Use Yoga as Medicine

Add this book to your collection, because with it you can use yoga to heal your mind, body, and spirit.

Get it now.

www.SFNonfictionBooks.com/Curing-Yoga

ABOUT SAM FURY

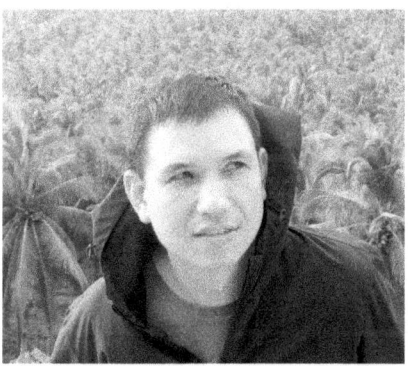

Sam Fury has had a passion for survival, evasion, resistance, and escape (SERE) training since he was a young boy growing up in Australia.

This led him to years of training and career experience in related subjects, including martial arts, military training, survival skills, outdoor sports, and sustainable living.

These days, Sam spends his time refining existing skills, gaining new skills, and sharing what he learns via the Survival Fitness Plan website.

www.SurvivalFitnessPlan.com

- amazon.com/author/samfury
- goodreads.com/SamFury
- facebook.com/AuthorSamFury
- instagram.com/AuthorSamFury
- youtube.com/SurvivalFitnessPlan

www.ingramcontent.com/pod-product-compliance
Lightning Source LLC
Chambersburg PA
CBHW070034040426
42333CB00040B/1672